MW00878761

YOU CAN TOO

MY JOURNEY TO BECOMING A NURSE ANESTHETIST

ANDREW S. FLOWERS, CRNA

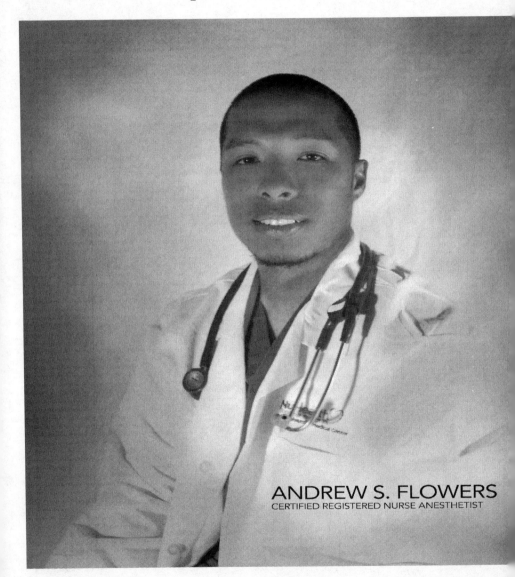

ANDREW S. FLOWERS
CERTIFIED REGISTERED NURSE ANESTHETIST

3

Editing done by : Brittany J. Mckeldin (bjmckeldin@gmail.com)

Cover done by: Olivia B. Mckeldin (oliviamckeldin@yahoo.com, bombshellstudiosnyc.com)

4

Preface

I remember how excited and enthusiastic I was when I first decided to pursue a career in healthcare. There was just one problem: I had no mentors that were in healthcare nor anyone to show me the steps I needed to take to get where I wanted to go. I had to learn by trial and error, and I spent countless hours doing research in my spare time to try and figure out the fastest way to become an advanced practice nurse. I eventually reached my goal in becoming a certified registered nurse anesthetist, but it took me about ten years from the time I made the decision to become one and about fifteen years after I graduated from high school. I always said to myself that if only I had a manual when I first started, to show me what to do to get to the finish line, it would not have taken me so long. This book is that blueprint for those who are interested in pursuing a career in nursing and want to accomplish it in the shortest amount of time. By laying out the steps in my journey to becoming a CRNA I provide encouragement, resources, and guidance to help you get through the extensive curriculum without wasting time. In this book you will find out more about who I am, what I experienced while

pursuing this career, and the lessons I've learned along the way.

Whether you want to be a nurse anesthetist, registered nurse,

physician assistant, nurse practitioner, physical therapist or any

other healthcare related professional, this book will help you

navigate the path to achieving your goal.

This book is dedicated to anyone who has a dream.

Acknowledgements:

There are so many people I want to thank for their contributions

to my success and accomplishments throughout my journey.

First, I would like to thank God for guiding me and giving me the opportunity to be where I am today. I also want to thank my fiancé, Rochelle, for holding me down and always being there for me, even when I was down and broke. Thank you to Tahj and Shanice for making me a better person, my father for raising me and showing me how to be man, my grandparents for guidance, and my aunts who continually show me unconditional love. More specifically, I am grateful for Auntie Shelly who always gives me good advice, Auntie Val for being there for me and giving me a roof over my head while in school, Aunt Jolynn for being direct and letting me have it straight, and Auntie Marcy for encouraging me. I also appreciate my uncles Artie and Harvey for helping me out when needed. I can't forget my cousins who gave me inspiration to push for more: Brittany, Olivia, Alexandria, Coryn, Lina, Daniel, Alex, and Samantha. I thank Annie Valentine, Professor Jenkins and Ms. Jenor who mentored me at Nassau Community College, and Professors Jennas and Bonbury who gave me a chance by accepting me into the CRNA program. Last but not least, I want to express gratitude to my friends who kept me grounded: Dewain, Henri, Michael, Sandro, Reggie, Tolani, Javier, and Glenn.

Table of Contents

10

Chapter 1
My Background

I'll start off by telling you a little about myself and where I am from. I am half Belizean and half Korean. I grew up in Queens Village, New York as a young kid. When I was about nine-years-old, my father and I moved from my grandmother's house to a town called Uniondale on Long Island in New York. Uniondale, a middle-class suburban neighborhood, is home to Hofstra University and the former home of the New York Islanders. Looking back, this was a great place to grow up, as it was a melting pot of hard-working, middle-class people from different races and ethnicities who took pride in their neighborhood. That's not to say that trouble was hard to find whether you were looking for it or not. As a kid growing up there, I found my fair share of trouble, but I was also fortunate enough to have family and friends around to set me straight.

My father is one of those people who did his best to kept me on the right track. He was a hard working man that raised me the best he could on his own. He worked two jobs to provide for us, which left me with a lot of unsupervised time alone. He was mild mannered but strong willed, and taught me many valuable lessons about life. He tried his best to give me balance. He taught me how to be a man and how to be a gentleman by example. I think we had a good time together while I was growing up. It was just the two of us against the world.

My father and mother separated when I was about 2-years-old, and I have only seen her once since then. From the time she left, she never kept in touch or reached out to me, but I wasn't mad at her. I became curious about who she was and I just wanted to know a little more about her and try to connect with the Korean side of me. So, I decided to look for her when I was about 20-years-old.

One day I found her address through some website and just decided to drive there. There were about 4 different addresses connected to her name. And all of them were only within approximately 20 minutes from where I lived. I expected her to at least live in another state since I haven't heard from her since I was 2-years-old. I started at the top of the list of addressed and worked my way down. I had no luck with the first three. I waited a few days to drive to last address because, in the early 2000s, getting directions wasn't as easy as putting the address into your smartphone and having Siri tell you exactly where to go. So, I had to go back home, go on MapQuest, print out the directions and hope that I didn't make a wrong turn on the way. I eventually found the last house on the list.

I pulled up to the house and knocked on the door, and my mother was the one who actually answered. The whole reunion went a little different than how I had imagined it unfolding in my head. I pictured us hugging right away and talking for hours and her apologizing that she never came for me. When she opened the door, I could hear people and kids in the background, but she wouldn't let me inside. I told her who I was and she said, "I have a new family and they don't know about you, so take my number and call me so we can talk." I took the number and left. I called that number she gave me a few times, and every time I called I would hear, in a thick Korean accent, "Nail salon. How can I help you?" I would ask for her but she never came to the phone. After several attempts I got the notion that she was brushing me off. I figured she did not want her new family to find out about me and I wasn't there to break up a happy home, so I decided to leave it alone. That time I went to her house was the last time I have seen or heard from my mother.

I am definitely more connected to the Belizean side (my father's side) of the family. Despite the situation with my mother, I still had a fruitful childhood where I did not want for anything. I always had a roof over my head and food in my stomach. I received an exponential amount of motherly love and discipline (aka head slapping) from my aunts and other strong women that accepted me as one of their own children , which made up for it.

I must say that there were a few pluses to growing up in a single-parent household being raised by my father. Since he worked a lot and there wasn't a woman in the house, I was forced to learn how to perform domestic duties from a young age. My father was a top chef when it came to making eggs, but unfortunately that was his only trick in the kitchen. My refrigerator never had fresh meat like whole chickens or anything you actually had to clean and cook from scratch. We would have no idea what to do with it anyway. Our fridge was filled with eggs, hot pockets, TV dinners, and other premade foods that came with microwave directions. If it could not be cooked with a microwave then it didn't belong in our house. Not having a mother around to cook forced me to learn how to make simple foods for myself as a child. If I was hungry and home alone, I had to learn quickly how to at least make basic foods like rice, eggs, and ramen. I also learned how to clean a house, do laundry, and do yard work. Thinking back, I'm glad I went through that because I see grown people today who can't do a load of laundry even if their lives depended on it. I believe my circumstances made me a little tougher and more independent growing up.

One thing about being half black and half Korean is that I did not look like anyone else around me. I definitely looked more asian than black back then. As an adult, I appreciate looking different, but as a kid it was difficult at times. As I mentioned before, I only know the Belizean (black) side of me and I grew up in a predominantly black neighborhood. At times it was hard to fit in when no one else looked like me. I remember when I would meet other kids for the first time, I'd tell them I was black and some would say things like, "You ain't black, you Chinese." Or I might start talking in slang from the neighborhood and people would ask, "Why you talking like that?" They would say that I was "acting black", but to me I wasn't acting; I was just being myself.

As a young kid I got into some fights because people would make fun of me looking Asian. I got made when they said things like duck sauce or when they pulled their eyes back to appear more Asian looking. There were times when people thought that my friends were my father's sons and I was the friend tagging along. There were some people who even thought

I was adopted. Kids can be cruel, but I eventually felt more comfortable in my own skin as I got older and I've learned to appreciate my uniqueness. Despite the ignorant people around me back then, I was fortunate enough to have good friends while growing up who saw past my physical features and accepted me for who I am.

The purpose of me sharing so much about my past is to say that your past does not dictate your future. The experiences you go through as a child, adolescent, and even a young adult shape you and give you skills you can use to your advantage. It's all about how you look at the situation. You can make unfortunate events in your life an excuse to be mediocre or you can use them to fuel you on your journey to greatness. I'm excited to share my journey with you.

Chapter 2
Get a Job or Go to School

High School to me at that time was more of a fashion show and a place I had to attend to play sports. By my senior year I only needed one class to graduate, yet I barely made it through. I was not motivated scholastically at all then, so I did just enough to get by. When it was time to graduate, I still did not have a plan of action in place. I barely gave college a thought and had no idea what kind of work I wanted to do or could do. I literally lived three blocks away from a prestigious university and I never once thought to walk over there and see what they had to offer. I walked around with this mindset that one day I would win the lottery or trip over a bag of money in the street, so there was really no need to prepare for my future.

After strolling in the house one summer day, my father said to me those infamous words no teenager wants to hear: "Get a job and help pay the bills or go to school. It's one or the other if you are going to live here."

The next day I found myself in the office of academic advisement at Nassau Community College not too far from where I lived. I decided to major in computer science mainly because my father received his degree in the same discipline. I had rationalized to myself that if there was something I couldn't figure out, I would just ask him for the answer.

I had no interest in computers what so ever and it showed. Coupled with my lethargic attitude towards school, my lack of knowledge on the subject was a setup for failure. By the end of my second semester I was placed on academic probation and facing being suspended from the school. I said to myself, "I work for minimum wage and I am about to get kicked out of community college. Where is my life headed?" I realized that something had to change quickly because community college was both my plan A and plan B. My options were running out.

If I could go back in time, I would have definitely taken school more seriously. There are options out there which can make you exempt from having to take unnecessary college courses, which would save you time and money. If you're interested in nursing, there are some high schools that offer courses that count towards college credits. If you're in highschool, consider taking advanced placement (AP) classes instead of taking the easy route your senior year. You can join organizations such as HOSA, an international student organization recognized by the U.S. Department of Education and the Health Science Education (HSE) Division of the

Association for Career and Technical Education (ACTE). You can

also take CLEP exams. The College Level Examination Program

(CLEP) is a group of standardized tests created and administered

by The College Board, the same organization that governs the

SAT. The CLEP exams assess college-level knowledge in thirty-

six subject areas and provide a mechanism for earning college

credits without taking college courses. You can find more

information at clep.collegeboard.org.

Chapter 3
The Lights Are Starting to Come On

I don't remember the exact day I found it or where I got it from, but I picked up a book called *Native Son* by Richard Wright, and I believe that one book changed my life forever. Normally, I avoided reading like the plague, but this time something told me to read this book. That book opened up my mind to literature and revealed to me a glimpse of the power that reading can have. It allowed me to exercise my imagination and use muscles in my brain I had never used before; it felt great! From then on I devoured books for breakfast, lunch and dinner. I read everything from *The Mis-education of the Negro* by Carter G. Woodson to *Rich Dad Poor Dad* by Robert Kiyosaki, and books from any other genre in between that I could get my hands on. I actually started requesting books as gifts for Christmas and birthdays. The more I read the more I felt like the light bulb in my head that flickered from time to time grew brighter and brighter.

My attitude made a 180-degree turn. I started believing in myself and in the fact that I could do anything that I put my mind to no matter how big the obstacle. My mindset went from how much could I get to how much can I give. I started to develop principles and discipline. I started to take a good look in the mirror and ask myself, "Are you wasting your talent or are you giving it your all? Is this all you want out of life or do you want to hang your hat as high as you can?" I noticed that, slowly but surely, everything around me was starting to change. My circle of friends, my speech, my attitude, my walk, and the music I listened to all changed. Most importantly, my grades started to improve.

Although I was turning my life around, I did encounter a few bumps in the road. I made some poor decisions that resulted in a couple of court dates; I believe this was the consequence of holding on to old friendships that I should have let go sooner. I spent countless hours in court and thousands of dollars on lawyer fees. Sometimes you have to pay to learn, and I definitely paid with money and time. Despite these setbacks, I maintained my focus on the bigger picture. I began utilizing my full potential and good things were happening, so I said to myself, "Why stop?" I now felt that the sky was the limit.

My advice to the youth preparing for college is to start reading at a young age. I regret not starting at an early age. If you don't like reading, start with any topic that interests you. For example, if you love basketball and like watching the highlights, like me, go on ESPN.com and read the article instead of watching it on television. I found reading to be a fundamental part of my mental growth, because it changed the way I view myself and the world. Information changes situations. I believe that knowledge is the new money, so go out there and get you some. The more knowledge you have, the better equipped you are to tackle any challenge you'll ever face. Look at Warren Buffet who in 2016 is #3 on the Forbes list of wealthiest people in the world worth over $70 billion; he is a big advocate of reading. According to him, he reads anywhere from 4 to 6 hours everyday. When Warren Buffett started his career in investments, he would read 600, 750, or 1,000 pages a day. Even now, he still spends about 80% of his day reading. He said, "I read 500 pages like this every day. That's how knowledge builds up, like compound interest." I'm not saying that we should all go out and read 1,000 pages everyday, but it's evident that reading does help one acquire knowledge that can allow for making quicker, informed decisions.

Chapter 4
My Real Estate "Empire"

Things were going well up until this point. I had a car; it was in the shop more than it was on the road, but it was still mine. I had a steady job at the Marriott washing dishes and my grades were in the B to A range. After taking a few biology courses and doing well in them, I realized I had a genuine interest in how the human body works. Then I got sidetracked by the bright lights surrounding what I thought was a get-rich-quick scheme.

I was still reading books whenever I could for leisure, and there was one book called *Rich Dad Poor Dad,* written by Robert Kiyosaki, that sparked a curiosity in me about real estate investing. I decided to look into finding more information about how and what it took to get started. After doing a little research online, I stumbled across something that said Robert Kiyosaki was going to give a lecture about real estate in Manhattan soon after I finished reading his book. I knew it had to be fate that I discovered his book and found out that he would be at a seminar near me around the same time. The book inspired me to become a real estate investor and to get on it ASAP.

I attended the seminar at the Jacob Javits center in Manhattan and walked out of it seeing dollar signs. This was prior to the real estate crash in 2007-2008, so there were no-money-down programs and all you really needed to qualify for a mortgage was a pulse. According to what I learned at the seminar, I met the criteria being that I didn't have any money, and I also didn't have any credit. So, I believed the hype and bought into the theory that I would become a millionaire by flipping and selling houses in no time. By the next weekend, I decided to give school a break and pursue real estate full-time.

When I told people at school about my plan, they tried to advise me against it. One classmate actually grabbed me by my shoulders, came about 3-inches from my face, and said very slowly, stressing every syllable, "Andrew, do not do it!" It was too late; all I could picture was myself wearing fancy suits and rolling up to my lawyer's office with my advisors talking about which blocks we should take over.

I took the next semester off, got a full time job as a car salesman in an attempt to make money to invest into purchasing houses and pursued my dreams to build my real estate empire. After months of hustling, I was never able to flip one house, and I was miserable working at the car dealership. I remember that it was winter and for most of the day my hands and feet were numb from showing people cars out on the lot. Even worse, I was a terrible salesman. I sold one car during my time there, and I had to split the commission with another salesman, because I could not close the deal by myself. After a few months, I handed in my resignation, even though I was probably close to getting axed anyway. At this point, I wound up being broker than ever, and I lost a semester in school. I'm not saying that buying houses for no money can't be done; I am just saying it didn't work for me at that time in my life.

I learned some valuable lessons that year. One being that sometimes people who love you and want good for you are giving you advice for a reason, because they can see something that you can't. It is good to be able to give advice but it's important to also allow yourself to receive advice. I learned that even though some people are able to achieve their goals in life by jumping in without a plan, it is vital for others to create well thought out, specific goals with deadlines. A clear and time-bound objective is more attainable and can help you achieve your dreams. What I did with my real estate fantasy was jump out in the middle of the ocean without a life vest, and I almost drowned.

Chapter 5
Back to School

I remembered that before taking a break from school, I was really interested in the sciences. So, I decided to pursue a career in the medical field. I wasn't sure of what I wanted to do, specifically, but I knew that was the direction I wanted to go in. I just couldn't picture myself being happy sitting in a cubicle and crunching numbers all day at a computer. I began contemplating becoming a medical doctor after reading a book called *The Pact*, by The Three Doctors and Lisa Frazier Page, which is about three childhood friends from the inner city area of New Jersey who made a pact that they would all go to medical school together in order to come back and help their communities in need of healthcare. That book resonated with me because the protagonists were also minorities who did not have the best start in life, but with a change in attitude they were able to fulfill their dreams.

Although I had chosen a career path, I had no idea how I was going to afford medical school to become a doctor. I looked into other, more practical options within the same field, and eventually found out what a physician assistant (PA) does. That job really interested me, so I decided that would be my goal.

Now back in school, I had to take Microbiology, which was a prerequisite for the PA program. Little did I know that the friendly talkative girl named Kelly who sat next to me would change the course of my life forever. By the end of the class, Kelly and I became good friends, and she told me that she was taking the class in order to apply for the nursing program at Adelphi University. She suggested to me that I, too, apply for the nursing program because, according to her, nursing was a good profession. At first, I actually scoffed at the idea because I thought that nursing was a profession for women only, and physician assistant sounded more manly. It didn't help that I just recently watched that movie *Meet the Fockers* in which Robert De Niro's character is making fun of Ben Stiller's character for being a male nurse. In addition to that, I thought that all nurses did was clean bed pans and dispense medication.

I found out shortly after that conversation with Kelly that there were more classes required for the PA program at the school I was interested in. I did, however, have all the

prerequisites necessary for the nursing program at Adelphi

University. It seemed like a no-brainer, so I applied and actually

got in, but I didn't get in right away. I say "actually" because I

couldn't believe it at the time. I was surprised because I sent my

application in after the deadline, and my GPA was slightly lower

than the required GPA they were asking for. But the way I was

able to get in was that I went to the school in person with my

transcripts in hand and asked to sit down with one of the

admissions counselors in the nursing building. I pleaded my

case that day. I had already spent almost six years at a two-year

college and I was desperately ready to move on. I told the

counselor that I would not let her down and she would not

regret allowing me into the program. It was around the summer

time and I told the admissions counselor that I knew my GPA

was below the requirement and showed her that my grades had

improved over time. I had bombed my first year in college so

badly that it was still bringing my GPA down to a 2.9 even

though I was consistently averaging a 3.5 and up after that year, and they required a 3.0 GPA. So, she made a deal with me. She said that I since I had completed all the prerequisites except for Pathophysiology, I could take the course over the summer and if I received at least a B+ she would let me into the accelerated nursing program the which started the following fall semester.

I was so excited to see the light at the end of the tunnel starting to shine through. I was so close but yet so far, because getting a B+ in that course was going to be tough, especially cramming four months worth of material into 6 weeks. That summer for me was all work and no play, but it was worth it because I got my B+ and was accepted into the nursing program at Adelphi University. After I got my acceptance letter, I started doing research on the nursing profession and liked what I was finding out.

Nurses had many options; they could work in almost any division of health care from labor and delivery to intensive care units to management. I also checked the salaries and they were more than I expected which didn't hurt to know. As I browsed the range of incomes, I noticed one title that exceeded the other nursing specialties, by far. That high-paying title was Certified Registered Nurse Anesthetist. After reading what the scope of practice was for that profession, coupled with the compensation, I had set a new goal; I would become a CRNA.

I have to be honest that the salary was the first thing that caught my attention about this profession, but after researching more about the scope of practice, I became more excited about what CRNAs do and the autonomy that they have at work. According to AANA's (American Association of Nurse Anesthetist)website, CRNAs are qualified to make independent judgments concerning all aspects of anesthesia care based on their education, licensure, and certification. It looked like achieving this new goal of mine was going to take years of planning, and I knew it was worth it. Every move I made from that day on was to get me closer to becoming a CRNA.

My advice for those who are figuring out what program of study to go into or which school to apply to, remember that the people who decide who gets in are people and not robots. This means that just because you may not look like a shining star on paper does not mean you can not get in. Many admissions departments look at the whole package and not just your GPA. So if you're not stellar on paper you might have to make them notice you by going to the school in-person and pleading your case. Show them how hungry you are for it!

Chapter 6
In the Nursing Program

I still remember my first day on campus. I thought to myself, "It took me over five years to finish a two-year degree program, but I still made it to the next level." It was a warm sunny day in September of 2005. I took a good look around, and to me it didn't matter that I wasn't on a large campus with all the luxuries that a bigger college or university might offer. I was just happy to be there. As a matter of fact, I realized that it was a good thing Adelphi wasn't a big "party school." The last thing I needed was to be tempted by partying all the time. If it was a party school, the title of this book might be *I Wonder What It's Like to Be a Nurse Anesthetist,* instead. With that said, I must admit that I envy those who can party hard and still have enough focus to do well in school.

The point is that when choosing a school, you have to know yourself. On top of that, you have to be honest with yourself about what works and what doesn't work for you. You have to ask yourself certain questions to figure out what kind of personality you have. Are you disciplined enough to go away to a big university where you will be surrounded by constant distractions and still be able to focus? Or are you more like me, where you get sidetracked very easily and there is no such thing as going out and having just one beer?

If you are more like me, it might be best for you to go to a local school until you mature enough to handle the independence that comes with being on your own, away from home. I suggest a community college or state school to keep the loans as low as possible. According to The College Board, the average cost of tuition and fees for the 2015–2016 school year was $32,405 at private colleges, more than three times the cost for state residents at public colleges, which was $9,410. So, don't feel bad if you did not get the opportunity to go to a large, well-known party school away from home; the smaller, quieter campus may help you graduate sooner, with better grades and less debt.

After my first few days of classes I said to myself, "This isn't so bad." Most of the classes were interesting and revolved around the sciences and nursing, which I started to love. Some of the courses I could have done without, such as nursing psychology because it was so difficult. But, the fact that 95% of the students were women made it more tolerable. I was fortunate enough to become friends with a nursing student named Latoya who turned out to be my anchor throughout the program by helping me stay organized and focused. We are still good friends to this day.

Along with taking regular lecture classes we all had to attend and perform well in clinicals. Nursing clinicals are supervised sessions in real world healthcare environments which allow nursing students to put their knowledge and skills to work. Clinicals are the nursing equivalent of internships for other disciplines and residencies for doctors, and they are a critical part of medical training as they give nursing students a chance to work with real patients. I had a love-hate relationship with clinicals. I hated the part about waking up early in the morning to be at the 7a.m. conference, but I loved interacting with patients and seeing how things I learned in class really worked in the field.

I found most of the classes to be difficult, yet manageable. However, there was one class that I almost failed, and no matter how hard I studied, I could not figure out how to approach the final test. That class was Psychiatric Nursing. I remember passing by the skin of my teeth only because my 74.5 rounded up to a 75.

If you're already in it or going to take it, don't feel bad if Psychiatric Nursing gives you trouble too. As far as I know, it's a challenging class for all nursing students. There is a book I wish I had known about when I took the class that you might find helpful called *Psychiatric Mental Health Nursing Success: A Q&A Review Applying Critical Thinking to Test Taking (Davis's Success)*, by Cathy Melfi Curtis and Audra Baker. Although I discovered this book after taking the class, I know it has been successful in helping other nursing students.

I learned a lot in clinicals. It gave me exposure to all the different units in the hospital. In the psychiatric rotation I learned that all of the patients in that unit are not "crazy," as society calls them. The majority of the patients I came in contact with functioned quite normally and seemed to live "normal" lives. They were in the psychiatric unit due to lacking coping skills after a traumatic life experience or because they might have been depressed and needed professional help to get through it. For example, I remember one patient who was very intelligent and who was actually a black belt in karate who could of probably killed me with his pinky if he wanted to. He was there for severe depression because his wife had passed away and that emotionally crushed him. So he voluntarily admitted himself so he would not harm himself.

Believe it or not, one of my favorite rotations was labor and delivery, which I thought I would probably dislike. On the contrary, I really enjoyed taking care of the newborn babies. Not only witnessing, but also assisting in the vaginal delivery of a baby is something you don't forget easily. Initially, there was yelling and screaming, followed by crying, then smiling and laughter. It was a crazy experience, to say the least.

To my surprise, school went by pretty fast, and in 2007 I graduated as a Bachelor in Nursing. I took a few weeks off to mentally reset and relax, and I landed a nursing job at the same hospital I worked in as a Comfort Squad Aide, which is similar to a Nurse Aide. I was able to work as a graduate nurse (GN) until I passed my boards. Fortunately, there are some hospitals that allow this.

For the future nurses, if you need to start working right away for financial reasons, ask the hospitals you are applying to if you can work as a GN until you pass your board exam. I recommend Feuer Nursing Review and Kaplan Test Prep's question bank to study for your board exam. You do not need to go overboard and buy a ton of different prep programs. Maintain your focus on one or two prep courses, and give yourself a few months of intense studying before you take it.

Chapter 7
Med-Surg

Med-Surg is short for medical-surgical unit, which was my first

placement as a registered nurse. This unit is usually where most

nurses start in their career. Med-surg is comprised of a little bit

of everything from patients with pneumonia to wound

infections. This is where I found out that nursing was exhausting

mentally and physically. I was responsible for taking care of

eight to twelve patients at once which meant administering

medication, conducting head-to-toe assessments, handling any complications, assisting with cleaning and feeding, and dealing with the family members of those eight to ten patients. On top of that, there were always miscellaneous tasks and unexpected issues that had to be dealt with as they came up.

Even though it was a lot of work, I loved med-surg, and I was pretty good at it. To be a nurse you have to wear many different hats throughout the day. You have to be part pharmacist, social worker, nutritionist, clinician, and psychiatrist. On any given day in the med-surg unit, you never knew what might happen. You could be faced with anything from having to perform cardiac life support on a patient to calling security because a schizophrenic patient climbed out of the window and made a run for it. I experienced a constant adrenaline rush that I could never get sitting behind a desk staring at a computer.

I soon found out that to become a nurse anesthetist, the majority of schools require applicants to have completed at least two years of critical care experience. When it comes to working in a critical care unit, most nurses have to crawl before they walk, meaning that they will probably have to do a year or two of med-surg before transferring to critical care.

A word of advice: Make sure you factor critical care experience into your time-line while planning your journey to becoming a CRNA. For those that have a great GPA and right amount of motivation, you may be able to bypass doing med-surg. In that case, what you want to do while you are completing your preceptorship towards the end of the nursing program is ask for special permission to do the preceptorship in a critical care unit; most students do it in a med-surg unit. This could possibly shave 1-3 years off of the time between getting your nursing degree and applying for an anesthesia program. A preceptorship is an intense clinical rotation in your last semester where you will be assigned to one unit and act as the primary nurse for an assigned number of patients. You have to meet a minimum number of hours on the unit, which usually takes a whole semester. In my opinion, you will only be able to leverage this rigorous requirement if you are an excellent student.

So, if you are granted permission to do your preceptorship in a critical care unit, at the end of that rotation you should ask the nurse manager at the same hospital if you can stay and work there after you graduate. This way, you can finish the critical care prerequisite for a CRNA program somewhere that you already know the staff and systems. If you are not able to get a job at the same hospital, the training still looks good on your résumé when applying elsewhere and you might be able to jump straight into a critical care unit at a different facility.

After a few years of experience with med-surg under my belt, it was time to transfer out to one of the critical care units. I procrastinated for a while due to several reasons: I had gotten comfortable with med-surg, I had a routine, and I had seniority. Deep down inside, I was apprehensive about stepping out of my comfort zone by transferring to a new unit and becoming the new guy again. Fortunately for me, one day I was working overtime in the emergency department with a calm and confident woman. I remembered that no matter what happened, this nurse never got nervous or frazzled. She was able to read EKG waveforms and knew other advanced nursing techniques that I was not trained on. By the end of the shift she said to me, "I like how you work, Andrew. I can tell you are a hard worker." Then she asked, "Would you be interested in working in the coronary care unit (CCU) with me, we need a few nurses.?" That whole day I was working next to the manager of the CCU and I didn't know it. A few weeks later she made some phone calls and I got the OK to transfer to the CCU which is a critical care unit.

From that experience, I learned to always be mindful of what comes out of my mouth and to keep my integrity by not taking short-cuts, because you never know who is watching.

Chapter 8
Anxiety

I had no idea what I had gotten myself into. The CCU was a different kind of "animal" compared to med-surg. The alarms ringing constantly from the monitors, ventilators and other machines keeping the patients alive were a shock to my senses. Each time an alarm went off, about every 5 seconds, I would jump up and make sure everything was all right. On the contrary, the seasoned CCU nurses were always calm even in the event of a real emergency. Training there was a definite struggle for me; I wasn't in Kansas anymore. This unit required all my energy and attention to survive each day. I had to learn to read EKG tracings and monitor ventilators in addition to other life-saving devices. I also learned how to administer advanced medications and intravenous drips, including how to titrate them. We usually had only two patients to take care of at a time, but these patients were much sicker than those I cared for in

med-surg. Some of the patients in CCU had about ten

intravenous drips at one time, they were mechanically

ventilated, septic, and hemorrhaging, along with other

comorbidities. I had to learn how to swim fast or I would've

quickly drowned there.

At first, it was so difficult for me that I suffered from anxiety,

which kept me up at all hours of the night. I would purposely

stay up late, until about 3 or 4 a.m., even if I had work the next

morning at 7a.m., because I thought the sooner I went to sleep

the sooner work would come. At that point, all I wanted to do

was go back to med-surg where I was comfortable, but I knew I

had to go through this in order to become a nurse anesthetist; so,

I pushed forward.

I began studying books on my own to become more familiar with

critical care terminology and best practices for treating the

patients. I picked up books like *Critical Care Nursing Made*

Incredibly Easy, by and other books that had big pictures to make

the information easier for me to understand. I was always the first in the unit and the last one to leave, because I was slower at

getting things done than the other nurses. Some of the nurses

even thought I had no business being there because I wasn't

ready. Fortunately, there were others who encouraged me to

keep going and made the work easier for me.

About six months in, I finally got the hang of it. The anxiety that I

used to get was gone, and I was able to enjoy being in the CCU

the same way that I enjoyed med-surg. I had become so

proficient working there that I would encourage the new nurses

who came in behind me. I told them, "I was in your shoes not

that long ago, and it will get better." I started to feel like an

actual clinician, and the new air of confidence I gained could be

seen in my walk. This confidence came from knowing that I

could take care of almost any patient in any department, no

matter how ill they were.

I remember one day, before working in the CCU, I was sent to

help out in the emergency room (ER) because they were really

busy. When I got there, the nurses asked me if could place IVs

and draw blood, but I didn't know how to do either at the time. I felt embarrassed when they questioned, "What good are you if you can't even do that?" and, "Why did you come here in the first place?" Now that I had experience in a CCU, when help was needed in the ER and they called for me, I was able take care of the most critically ill patients. This time, instead of being looked at like I was useless, the nurses thanked and praised me for coming to help.

After about a year and a half in the CCU, I was pretty comfortable, and I had a routine down. The CRNA program I wanted to apply to required that I have at least 2 years of intensive care training, called ICU for short in the medical world, however, they would accept a year of CCU experience toward that. This meant that I would have to transfer to the ICU (intensive care unit) within the same hospital I was currently working or go to another hospital for at least 1 year, so that I could put ICU training on my application. Once again I was faced with having to move on right after adapting and gaining some seniority within the unit. Although this was a bit of a downer, I reminded myself of the big picture and I had to do what I had to

do in order to get there.

After a few days of looking online for a job I saw that Columbia

Presbyterian hospital in New York City had a position available

in the Medical ICU (MICU), so I applied, and after an interview I

was offered a position. I put my two weeks in at CCU and kept it

moving.

Chapter 9
The Big Leagues

Once again, I had no idea what I had gotten myself into. In my head I thought that the transition from the CCU to the MICU would be easy; I was wrong. The CCU at a smaller community hospital could not be compared to an ICU at a large, prestigious city hospital like Columbia. After only a few days on the unit, that old friend – anxiety – came creeping back in. I was shell-shocked again and experienced the same feelings I had when I transferred from med-surg to CCU.

It was like reliving a nightmare. The patients were extremely sick, and the pace was faster than the CCU. I had to learn how to chart on a computer system, which was new to me coming from paper charting. I also had to quickly learn how to manage new machines that I had never been exposed to before or even knew existed. On top of that, I was the new guy again and it sucked. I had to prove myself all over again, and in nursing if you make a visible mistake, you will be branded as a screw-up for life. These guys did not let anyone die; they had all kinds of machines: ECMO*, CVVHD*, Liver dialysis machines, and LVAD's* – things that I only read about in books. We even had to do our own

dialysis. Now it made sense to me why the school wanted at least

1 year of additional ICU experience, it was a big difference

between my CCU at a community hospital and this MICU.

It took me a while to catch on to the fast pace and new

technology, but I eventually did, just as I had previously adjusted

to life in the CCU. After about six months, I became comfortable

and the anxiety faded. I had proven myself to the staff and I

could just go to work and enjoy what I was doing again.

Besides everything going on inside the unit, I had to also get

used to the long daily commute. I went from driving 5 minutes

to work to over an hour-long trip. On top of that, I had to start

on the night shift, which my body had to adjust to. I was a

walking zombie on my days off, but I kept going as I said to

myself, "Whatever I have to do to get into that CRNA program, I

will do."

I worked in the MICU at Columbia Presbyterian for about 3 years

save up some money because I knew that most CRNA programs

were full time and they did not allow you to work while in the program. Immediately when I started working as a nurse I was a little careless with my money., I spent a lot of my money on cars, clothes, and girls, and the rest I wasted. This was the mentality I had the first few years. While I was working at Columbia, I still had fun and traveled every couple of months, but I became more disciplined with my money and it was paying off.

My bank account was stacking up and I was getting closer to being able to apply to the CRNA program. I worked my ass off and put in as much overtime as possible to keep adding to my bank account. I downgraded the car that I paid about $400/month for once my lease was up and bought an old 2000 Cadillac Deville for about $3000 cash; I drove that car until the wheels fell off. I loved that car, by the way. It was like riding on clouds and I could fit about 5 bodies in the trunk. I was tempted at times to get a new car and floss (show off), but I had to constantly remind myself that "flossing" would not get me to my goal. When it came to my wardrobe, I rarely bought clothes at full price anymore. However, I did have a weak spot – some would call it an addiction – for Polo Ralph Lauren, so I would go into the store and head straight for the clearance rack to get my fix every once in a while.

I believe what helped me save the most was that I opened two separate bank accounts. I had it set up so that every paycheck was split, with a set amount of money being automatically transferred to my savings account while the rest went into my checking. This way I could see exactly how much I was saving and keep track of the progress towards my target.

This is for you future CRNA students who know that sometimes you have to sacrifice what you're used to for something better in the end. I know it's hard to go from eating at fancy restaurants, wearing new clothes, and driving a nice car to go to back to sacrificing, but you have to give up good to be great.

Chapter 10

It's Now or Never

"Now it's time to stop talking about it and be about it," I thought; and I had the courage to actually be about it. I started to put my application for the CRNA program together, but there was still one part that made me nervous. For some reason I was scared that no one would want to write me a recommendation letter because they didn't think I was a good candidate or they just didn't have the time. Despite my fear, I knew it had to be done, so I asked one of the Nurse Practitioners on the unit indirectly if she knew anybody that wouldn't mind writing a recommendation letter for me for school. To my surprise she said "I would love to write one for you if you want." Well, that wasn't so hard! And just like that I had more confidence to finish up my application and send it out.

I made sure all my T's were crossed and I's were dotted, sent my application out, and I said a prayer. I was called in for an interview a few weeks later and thought I made it to the next step. I was very nervous sitting in the waiting room for my turn to be interviewed. There were about six other people waiting who looked confident and poised, and I thought, "Am I the only one that's nervous here?" because the rest of them were making small talk and cracking jokes amongst one another while I was sitting there praying the whole time. I read a bible verse on my phone that calmed me down and gave me reassurance and confidence. Philippians 4:13 states, "I can do all things through Christ which strengthens me." As my name was called I took a deep breath and said to myself, "Here goes nothing."

The interview was pretty intense. I had to sit directly across the table from the Dean and two other professors. I was greeted with warm smiles initially that quickly turned into three stone cold faces. Once the poker faces came on it was straight to business. There were no warm-up questions to get the juices flowing. From the jump, they began to give me difficult clinical scenarios and asked how I would respond to them. They did not want vague responses; they wanted detailed answers, and every answer I gave them would set up the next question they threw at me. I tried to read their faces to get some reassurance that I was on the right track, but their emotion-less faces gave me no clues that I was telling them what they wanted to hear, not even a head bob. I gave them the best answers I could, and if I didn't know something I just told them I didn't know. Before I knew it the interview was over and what seemed like an eternity was really only about fifteen minutes.

A few months later I pulled up to my house and I saw a large yellow envelope in the mailbox. "It must be my acceptance letter," I thought as I ran towards the mailbox and ripped open the letter. It stated: Dear Mr. Flowers, thank you for your application to the program. Unfortunately, you were not selected for a seat in the program, but you were placed on the alternate list and if a seat opens up, your name will be at the top of the list. I was disappointed but I was still hopeful, because I know that as long as I was on the alternate list there was a chance, and that meant I must have said something right in the interview. I also felt better knowing that they only accepted 12 students a year out of about 100 applicants.

The first day of school passed and I still did not receive a call. I was a little bummed, but I knew there was always next year. So, I waited patiently and reapplied when it was time, and I played the waiting game again. A few months later I was called for an interview and once again they got straight to business, just like the first time. I felt pretty good afterwards and once again I left it all on the table. Months went by and I did not hear any word, I did not even receive an alternate list letter. I started to think that I should start applying to other schools or even change my goal. Feelings of doubt began creeping in and I was losing confidence and motivation.

Then, all of a sudden, just about a month before the first day of class would start I got a phone call from the Dean offering me a seat in the program. My response was, "Absolutely! Sir, thank you for the opportunity." I really wanted to say, "Hell yeah brother! What do you think? It's about time you called!" But I had to keep it professional. I almost didn't think the phone call was real, and that it was all part of my imagination. I got down on my knees and thanked God right after I hung up the phone. Once I received an actual acceptance letter in mail it started to feel real.

****

****

For those looking to become CRNAs, here are a few websites that helped me narrow down the programs I wanted to apply to:

1) http://www.all-crna-schools.com - This is a great website that breaks down all the programs by state. It tells you everything from tuition costs to the prerequisites needed to get

in. Not all data is completely up to date, so you should verify with the school itself for more accurate information.

2) http://www.diversitycrna.org - The mission of the **Diversity in Nurse Anesthesia Mentorship Program** is to inform, empower and mentor underserved and diverse populations with information to prepare for a successful career in Nurse Anesthesia. I personally know several people who this program has helped with applying to CRNA programs.

****

When it comes to applying, I've learned that it's important to be seen as much as possible by the faculty and other members of the program (i.e. professors, Dean, and current students. If they become familiar with your name and face, it can only benefit you. Find out if the program your interested in offers information sessions, local mixers, or any other events where you can meet people.

Chapter 11
In the Program

On the first day of class, I was nervous, but I felt a little relieved

when I saw a familiar face. It was a guy named Tolani who I used

to work with at Columbia Medical Center. We both knew the

other had applied, but we didn't know that we both got in. We clicked right away. There was another face there that I recognized from the waiting room at my second interview. "That's right! The guy from California," I thought. I remembered him being relaxed and calm, so relaxed that he would not stop talking as we waited to be called in. Eventually, I had to excuse myself from the room because I couldn't focus. The talkative guy was Javier, and we actually became really tight throughout the program. Both Tolani and Javier became like my brothers by the end of the program along with my other classmates.

The first day of class was similar to the interview process, intense. The first day of class we got drilled about the anatomy of the airway. We were told to stand in a circle while the professor stood in the middle and pointed to one of us at random to answer each question. This first exercise set the tone for most of the program from that day forward. A few weeks in I began to realize why most programs either don't allow you to work or highly recommend not working at the same time you're taking classes. Not only was the workload huge, but also the subjects we were reading about were difficult to understand. The books were written in English, but at times the language of anesthesia was like reading French to me. I would read something about ten times and still have no idea what I just read. Most of my classmates and I were literally in the library an average of 14-16 hours a day. After the first few weeks, just like when I had transferred from unit to unit in the hospital, I asked what the hell I had gotten myself into? I really wasn't sure if I was going to make it through. I was already studying as much as I could and but I still wasn't really getting it. Even my boy Javier had thoughts of going back to California, because the CRNA program was extremely draining on us, mentally, emotionally, and physically. I thought to myself, "Was my life really that bad before as a floor nurse? I mean, I had a good salary, seniority, vacation time, and was somewhat comfortable."

In the beginning, there was some competition amongst us. We all thought that we could get through this program without any help, study alone in a corner somewhere and impress each other with how easy the information was. I quickly learned that even if you are intellectually gifted and come in with a 4.0 GPA, you can only survive by working together with your classmates. We all learned that, and after a few months we realized that we needed each other to make it through.

Over time, we slowly started to recognize each person's strengths and weaknesses, and we allocated assignments to one another based on who was good at what. For example, there was a course we took during our first semester called Physics in Anesthesia, and yes it was even harder than it sounds. The rest of us were weak in math and we were struggling in this class, but we realized that it came easy to Ermias, a guy who was originally from a country called Eritrea in Africa. He was a genius when it came to math. I remember a time when the professor could not quite explain how he arrived at a certain answer and Ermias stepped in to explain it. So, several times a week Ermias would get everybody together in an empty classroom and tutor us on the latest assignment. Because of this, we all called him Professor E. Although Ermias was great at math, his weakness was public speaking. So for any group assignment we had that required a presentation, we would delegate the speaking part to someone else that was good in front of an audience.

My boy Javier, the designated speaker most of the time, had several gifts; one was the gift of making us laugh. This was vital to our survival because there were so many tense and serious moments throughout the program that he made going to the library and being in class more tolerable. He also had a lot of life experience and was someone who you could go to for advice. He had seen and done it all at a young age; we joked that he was in his mid 30's going on 60.

Going back to Tolani, he had great leadership skills. We elected him class president because he always had the group's best interest in mind and set a great example of how to work hard. I think he pushed all of us to give a little more when we thought we couldn't. His motto was "PUSH." When any of us wanted to throw in the towel, he would say, "Come on, PUSH!" Persist Until Something Happens. And Saka who was never scared to challenge the status quo, he was a great problem solver and love to question why things were done a certain way. If we hadn't

swallowed our pride and gotten over our egos, I believe it would
have been almost impossible to pass. Once we left ourselves
vulnerable and allowed people to see our weaknesses, it was
easier for all of us to admit when we didn't understand
something. This allowed to the group to become closer and like
a family. It was a good thing we got along, because we were
together with each other more than we were with our own
families.

For the future students you have to prepare yourself mentally
that if you are accepted into a program it will be one of the
hardest things you will ever do. For the first year and a half it
will consume your life. You will have no personal life. Forget
about birthdays, weddings, and vacations. You might even have
to miss a few funerals. For the first year, your significant other
will be your textbook. It is important that you talk to your
family, friends, spouse, fiancé, boyfriend or girlfriend to let them
know you will be missing in action for a while and to ask for
their patience and support. At the time, my girlfriend Rochelle,
who is now my fiancé, played a vital role in me surviving the

program. She was my rock that kept me stable, and she supported me through the whole process. I don't know if I could have made it if it wasn't for her patience and words of encouragement, and that delicious home cooked food.

Chapter 12

How Could Things Be Worse?

Just when I thought it couldn't get any tougher, we were told we would be starting our clinical rotation. This is what we had prepared for over a year and a half, but we were still nervous. We heard horror stories of students from the past who had made some big mistakes in their clinical rotation, and no one wanted to be that person that would live in infamy as and example of what not to do. Our fate was to be decided by pieces of paper with the hospital names that we had to randomly pick out of a hat. This would tell us which hospital we would be starting the rotation at. I didn't care which hospital I got, as long as it wasn't Kings County Hospital in Flatbush, Brooklyn. It was a good hospital, but it had a reputation of being tough on the students. And then there was the infamous Dr. Alexis who was known to be the toughest. A few students pull out names and get lucky by picking the hospitals they wanted. It was my turn next. I hoped that their good luck would rub off on me. I stepped up and pulled a small piece of rolled up paper out of the hat and opened it. It said "Kings County Hospital." Anxiety took over fast, but immediately went away when my boy Tolani pulled out Kings County, too. My thought was, "At least I won't have to suffer alone."

After all the fuss, Kings County wound up being the best place for me to start. It's a trauma 1 hospital so they get everything from gun shot wounds to liver resections. We had a good amount of cases a day and were allowed to do a lot. Luckily, the CRNAs and Anesthesiologists were patient with us and were willing to teach us what they learned over the years.

Although it was better than I anticipated, I didn't think it was so great initially. We would be given our assigned cases the night before and we had to be prepared to report on them early the next morning during rounds at 7 a.m. To get to the hospital took me an hour, so that meant I was up around 4:45 a.m. to beat rush hour and get there on time everyday. One of the Anesthesiologists, usually Dr. Alexis, would randomly pick any student to present on his or her case. You had to give them everything from how you were going to put that patient to sleep, how you would keep the patient asleep, and how you would wake the patient up. You also had to go over all of that individual's medical problems and diseases and discuss how it would affect the patient and the anesthesia plan. They could ask you at any given time about any of your patients. And if you showed up unprepared, Dr. Alexis would be all over you. It was nightmare any time I looked up a patient the night before, and he or she had every known comorbidity or disease known to man. I would be up for hours after clinical preparing for my report on that one patient. Sometimes I wouldn't be done until 1 or 2 a.m. in the morning and then be up at 4:45 a.m. Sleep was a luxury at this moment in my life. The worse part was not being called on after all those hours of preparation. My classmates and I were all going through similar situations at different hospitals, all while taking our regular classes.

Dr. Alexis was actually great to work with. I remember trying to stay out of her sight at all costs at first. She was tough, but fair. She just wanted every student that came to Kings County to be better clinicians in the end. By the time Tolani and I were done there, we were different people. They shaped and molded us into sharper stronger students. After leaving the County we felt comfortable rotating anywhere we were placed. We knew it was a blessing having gone to Kings County because we heard from other students at different hospitals that they weren't getting a good clinical experience. Some of the students were initially happy where they were because no one challenged or tested them, but because of that they weren't at the same level as Tolani and I.

For the future CRNA students, don't believe everything you hear about other people. Sometimes what might seem like an unfair situation may actually be the best situation for you. As long as you do your part and come prepared there is nothing anybody can say negatively about you. Also, be humble and be like a sponge, absorb everything. Nobody likes a know-it-all, and trust me there is no way you will ever know it all.

Chapter 13
The Last Year

I finally started to get the hang of this anesthesia thing and felt

good walking into clinical sites. Most of the rotation sights

would assign me to a room alone to manage the cases, and that

made me feel that they trusted me and saw that my skills were improving. It was exciting to be doing procedures such as placing epidurals, A-lines, and central lines and also to be performing intubation on people. One technique that I had trouble improving on was spinals. A spinal is a technique where you administer medication to a patient into the spinal canal through their back that makes them numb from the stomach area down to the legs. This allows the patient to be awake while feeling nothing down below. These are good for procedures like C-sections or most surgeries in the lower portion of the body, like knee surgeries. Whenever I had to do a spinal, I could not find the right spot to save my life! For months and months I tried but was unsuccessful. Even though I was frustrated with myself I thought, "If I keep practicing I will eventually get it." I chased down spinals like my life depended on it. Whenever I saw a room with a patient that needed one, whether or not it was my assigned room, I always asked if I could do it. It got to the point where it was known amongst the staff that I wanted all the spinals. So, instead of me having to chase them down, people came to find me to do them. Eventually I got better at them and started to find the right spot on each patient's back.

For the future CRNA students, remember this: If you're not good at something at first just keep trying and don't worry about how you look to other people. There are two things in life you cannot do at the same time, i.e. look good and learn. You have to sacrifice one or the other. And trust me, I know I looked liked a clumsy fool trying to find that spot at first, but I didn't care, because in the end you can't focus on looking good in front of your teachers and focus on learning at the same time.

Looking back at my time in the CRNA program, the last year was a little easier due to the fact that the classes were less intense and there were fewer of them to take. As you can tell from previous chapters, the first year was the hardest, but I made it through. When compared to the first, the second year was more tolerable. We pretty much just went to clinical Monday through Saturday, except for one day, which would be spent in class. It was definitely more manageable at that point, but still tiring and frustrating at times. By the second year most of us were getting more comfortable with administering anesthesia and we were learning more and more with every day that went by.

During the second year of the program we were allowed to take some trips to anesthesia conferences around the country. We even had the opportunity to go to Washington D.C. to lobby for CRNA rights and privileges and help continue the growth of our practice. While we were there, I couldn't help but think about how I went from a lost kid, hustling in the streets to make a dollar, to sitting down and talking to senators and delegates in the nations capital. After every trip I would always come back home with a different perspective on life and the angle from which I viewed the world always got a little wider.

I had some great teachers along the way, and of course, I also had some that weren't the most pleasant to be around and who made the days seem longer. There were those that would give me so much confidence, which made going to clinical a blast. Even if one of the students made a mistake, they wouldn't make us feel bad about it. On the other hand, the ones that made the days seem longer would have me so nervous I would be paralyzed from fear of even blinking the wrong way. God forbid any of us made a mistake, they would verbally assault the culprit until he felt sorry for even being born.

What made things harder was my savings dwindling down, and we were not getting paid at these rotations.

It took me about ten years from the first time I decided to become a CRNA to actually become one. Even with all the ups and downs and frustrations, I know it was all worth it. Although it felt as if the rest of the world had passed me by for a few years, and at the end of the program I was broke and tired, I have no regrets. Putting myself in this position allowed me to see how much pain I could endure and made me a stronger person at the end of it. It allowed me to see who my true friends and family really are and who would be there to help if I needed it.

I believe we are all given opportunities when we are responsible and mature enough to handle them. It was probably a good thing that I had to wait a little longer to get in the program due to that fact I still had some growing up to do mentally. I probably wouldn't have nurtured, protected and respected this journey so much if it had come so easy to me. One important thing the program did was snap me out of the spending sprees I used to go on and the reckless way I managed my money. It also made me realize what's really important in my life, which are my family and friends and not so much materialistic things.

Expensive things are nice to have also, don't get me wrong, and there is no harm in buying those things if you can afford them. All I'm saying is it made me see what the differences are between necessities and wants.

My main point is that if you have a goal you want to reach that's worth working for, it is not going to be easy. There will be setbacks and disappointments along the way. Some of you might have it a little harder than others depending on your circumstances, but I wrote this story to let those who have a vision and a dream know even though you may not have had the best start, how you finish is what matters. Point blank, if you have a dream go chase that shit.

Hopefully in a few years I will have another book out called *From CRNA to Real Estate Developer*. It might take another ten years but I'll get there eventually.

If you have questions I can be reached at

andrewsflowers82@gmail.com

Appendix A - Appendix A - Miscellaneous Resources That Gave Me Motivation

Quotes:

-"With struggle there is no progress" Frederick Douglas

-"When you want to succeed as bad as you want to breathe then you will be successful" Dr. Eric Thomas (the hip hop preacher)

Music: Nas, Tupac, The Roots

Appendix B - Medical Terms Glossary (* throughout)

ECMO- extracorporeal membrane oxygenation (ECMO). The purpose of ECMO is to allow time for intrinsic recovery of the lungs and heart; a standard cardiopulmonary bypass provides support during various types of cardiac surgical procedures.

CVVHD- Continuous veno-venous hemofiltration (CVVH) was designed as a renal replacement therapy for patients with acute renal failure. It is often chosen over intermittent hemodialysis when blood pressure instability is a problem, and CVVH is generally more efficient than peritoneal dialysis.

LVAD- A left ventricular assist device (LVAD) is a pump that we use for patients who have reached end-stage heart failure. We surgically implant the LVAD, a battery-operated, mechanical pump, which then helps the left ventricle (main pumping chamber of the heart) pump blood to the rest of the body.

Epidural- Epidural anesthesia is the injection of a numbing medicine into the space around the spinal nerves in the lower back. It numbs the area above and below the point of injection and allows you to remain awake during the delivery. It can be used for either a vaginal birth or a cesarean delivery (C-section).

Spinal- anesthetic medicine is injected using a much smaller needle than an epidural needle, directly into the cerebrospinal fluid that surrounds the spinal cord.

Central line - A central venous catheter, also called a central line, is a long, thin, flexible tube used to give medicines, fluids, nutrients, or blood products over a long period of time, usually several weeks or more.

A-line- An arterial line (also art-line or a-line) is a thin catheter inserted into an artery. It is most commonly used in intensive care medicine and anesthesia to monitor blood pressure directly and in real-time (rather than by intermittent and indirect measurement) and to obtain samples for arterial blood gas analysis.

Intubation- Tracheal intubation, usually simply referred to as intubation, is the placement of a flexible plastic tube into the trachea (windpipe) to maintain an open airway or to serve as a conduit through which to administer certain drugs.

Regional Block - Regional anesthesia is the use of local anesthetics to block sensations of pain from a large area of the body, such as an arm or leg or the abdomen. Regional anesthesia allows a procedure to be done on a region of the body without your being unconscious.

36267738R00051

Made in the USA
San Bernardino, CA
19 May 2019